Wala BEN KRIDIS
Afef KHANFIR

Brain metastases of breast cancer

Wala BEN KRIDIS
Afef KHANFIR

Brain metastases of breast cancer

Anatomoclinical and therapeutic characteristics

ScienciaScripts

Cover image: www.ingimage.com

This book is a translation from the original published under ISBN 978-620-3-44872-6.

Publisher:
Sciencia Scripts
is a trademark of
Dodo Books Indian Ocean Ltd. and OmniScriptum S.R.L publishing group

120 High Road, East Finchley, London, N2 9ED, United Kingdom
Str. Armeneasca 28/1, office 1, Chisinau MD-2012, Republic of Moldova, Europe
Printed at: see last page
ISBN: 978-620-5-73161-1

BRAIN METASTASES OF BREAST CANCER

ANATOMOCLINICAL AND THERAPEUTIC

CHARACTERISTICS WALA BEN KRIDIS*, AFEF KHANFIR

Dr. Wala BEN KRIDIS is Associate Professor at the Faculty of Medicine of Sfax (Tunisia).

Graduate in medical carcinology (MD)
Diploma in biological sciences (PhD)
Master of Clinical Research in Medical Sciences
Certificate of Additional Studies in Fundamental Education
Certificate of complementary studies in ENT carcinology and cervicofacial surgery

Certificate of complementary studies Tumors of the locomotor system
Certificate of complementary studies in medical English
Reviewer in Journal of international medical research, Radiation Oncology, Therapeutic Advances in Medical Oncology, Future oncology, Breast disease...

Editor in international journal of prostate cancer
Review Editor in Frontiers in oncology

walabenkridis@yahoo.fr

SUMMARY

Breast cancer is the first cancer of women in the world and in Tunisia with an incidence of 46.3 and 37.8 cases / 100 000 inhabitants per year respectively.

It is the second cause of cancer mortality in women in Tunisia with 17 deaths / 100 000 inhabitants per year.

The management of metastatic breast cancer has undergone several advances over the past decades resulting in improved patient survival. However, 15 to 30% of patients will develop brain metastases (BM) during the course of their disease.

They can occur synchronously (at the time of diagnosis of the primary cancer) or metachronously (after 6 months of the end of the primary cancer treatment).

The management of CD is multidisciplinary, involving neurologists, neurosurgeons, radiologists, radiation oncologists, medical oncologists and pathologists.

Radiation therapy (RT) is one of the mainstays of CD treatment and has long been the standard treatment with its different modalities.

The place of surgery is discussed according to the operability and the resectability of metastases, as well as systemic disease status.Systemic treatment can be based on chemotherapy, hormone therapy and targeted therapy and depends on the terrain, molecular classification and previously prescribed treatments.

Keywords: breast cancer, brain metastases, epidemiology, clinical, treatment

1- EPIDEMIOLOGY

CD due to breast cancer constitutes 15-20% of the etiologies of secondary brain lesions[1, 2 ,3]. It is the second most frequent etiology, after lung cancer, of CD [4, 5 ,6]. Their incidence has been increasing in recent years due to the development of therapeutic management of breast cancer, the improvement of systemic disease control, the increase in patient survival and the performance of new imaging techniques [6].

The incidence of CD in breast cancer is estimated to be 15-20 % and reaches 30% in autopsy series [7-9]. It was more observed in the HR-negative, Her2-overexpressed and triple-negative subgroups (20-30%) [10-12].

CD in breast cancer occurs at an earlier age than in other primary sites [6], which is consistent with the results of our series. In a study by DeLesoet al, who collected 274 patients with brain metastatic breast cancer, the age of onset was 53 years[13]. Benna et al found, in a study of 139 patients treated for MC, a mean age of onset of 49 years in the MC subgroup secondary to breast carcinoma[14].

The onset of CD is often late. It is metachronous in more than 80% of cases and occurs after the visceral and/or bone progression of disease[15]. The low percentage of patients with synchronous CD may be explained by an underestimation of the actual number of cases where the disease was initially metastatic to the brain, as brain imaging is not part of the initial routine work-up of the disease[16]. Alternatively, the central nervous system may be the only site of recurrence of metastatic disease. De Leso et al found in his series 9.5% of patients with only MC [13].

In the literature, brain-only metastatic disease was most often observed in the Her overexpressed subgroup since the introduction of targeted therapies that improved the control of metastatic disease in other metastatic sites but their action on the brain was less marked due to their poor passage through the blood-brain barrier[17].

HER2 overexpression is a risk factor for brain metastasis. In a Canadian study, the incidence of brain metastases as the first site of metastatic relapse was 0.4% for tumors without HER2 overexpression and 9% for tumors with HER2 overexpression (12). The US RegistHER registry recorded 1,023 patients treated for HER2-overexpressing breast cancer between December 2003 and February 2006. Metastatic disease was found in 768 of them. One third of the metastatic patients had brain progression. The median time to onset of brain metastases. Breast tumors developed in patients with BRCA1 mutations are also frequently complicated by brain metastasis. A retrospective series from the Gustave-Roussy Institute (Villejuif) analyzed the evolution of 70 patients with a BRCA1 mutation. Fifteen patients had metastatic disease, including 10 (67%) with secondary cerebral localizations. The median time to onset of these brain metastases from the first metastatic event was 7.8 months. This can be explained by the triple-negative status frequently encountered in BRCA-mutated breast cancer.

2. CLINICAL FEATURES

The clinical presentation of CD in breast cancer does not differ from its presentation in other primary diseases. It is a polymorphic subacute neurological symptomatology that depends essentially on the location of the metastases.Symptoms are dominated by isolated headaches, signs intracranial hypertension (ICHT), focal neurological deficits, and seizures, behavioral and language disorders and several other neurological clinical manifestations[18].

In a study by Saha et al, who collected 72 patients treated for CD, headache was the most frequent reason (66%) followed by vomiting (54%) and focal neurological deficits (39%)[19].

3. CONTRIBUTION OF IMAGING

The development of imaging techniques has led to improved detection of CDs. The advent of multimodal imaging has allowed a better characterization of CDs. The diagnosis of single CDs has regressed in recent decades in favor of multiple brain lesions. This is partly explained by the performance of MRI with its different sequences (diffusion, perfusion, spectroscopy...) and the injection of Gadolinium, which is the examination of choice in the diagnosis of brain lesions[6]. In the study published by Saha et al, MC were multiple in 77%[19]. Spectroscopy is an interesting MRI sequence in tumor pathology. It consists in quantifying the different molecules present in the tissues, thanks to their different resonance frequency, after removing the signal from the l' water.

The molecules studied are N-Acetyl Aspartate (NAA): which is a neuronal marker that decreases in case of suffering and neuronal death, the Choline which increases during membrane synthesis and catabolism and cell proliferation and inflammation and Lactate which is not visible in the physiological state and increases during anaerobic metabolism[20].

Thus at the level of a tumor lesion there is a decrease in NAA and an increase in peak choline and lipids.

Cerebral CT still has a place in the diagnosis of CD, despite a false-negative rate of 11%, given its availability and easier access, especially in emergency situations. On CT, metastases have the same or slightly lower density than the brain parenchyma (Figure 1, 2), and are hyperdense when they are the site of hemorrhagic phenomena[21].

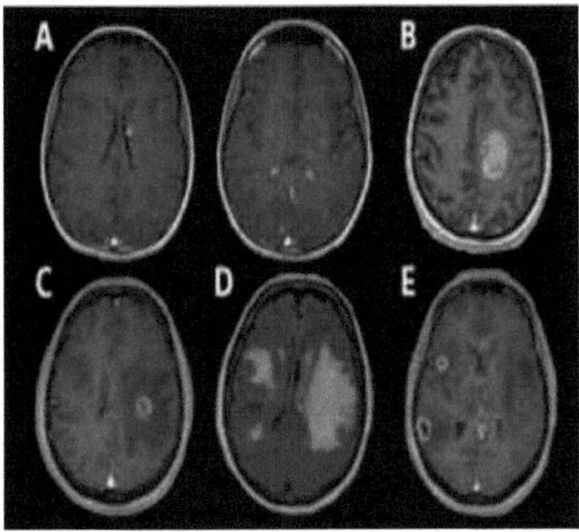

Figure 1: Multiple brain metastases from breast cancer creating a metastatic miliary (A). Note the predominance at the white matter-gray matter junction. Single hemorrhagic metastasis (B, C). Note the very marked cerebral edema (D) and the typical annular contrast (E).

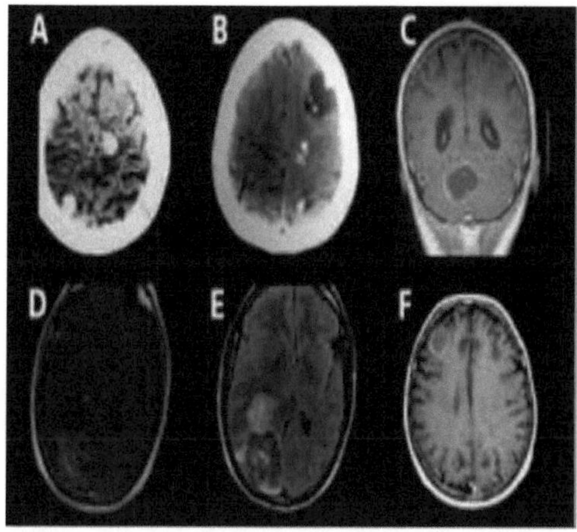

Figure 2: Spontaneously hemorrhagic metastases on non-injected CT scan(A). Calcified metastases (B). Cystic cerebellar metastasis (C). Single metastasis (D, E). Note however the Flair hyposignal aspect (E). Thin-walled cystic metastasis that may suggest an abscess (F)

On MRI, lesions in T1 sequence have a signal identical to the gray matter or slightly lower and in T2 sequence are hypersignal (Figure 3) [19].

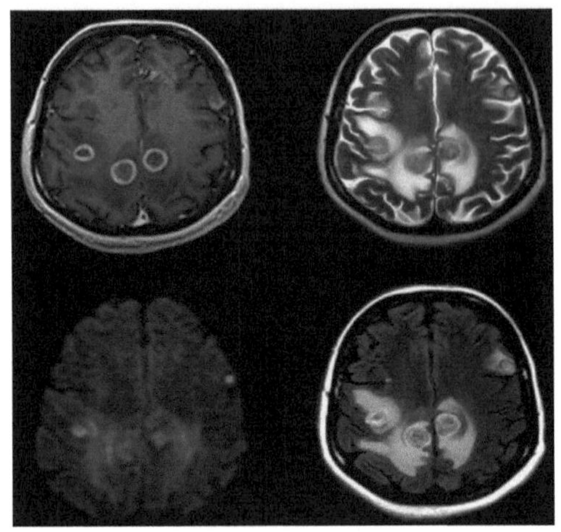

Figure 3: Brain metastases

4. THERAPEUTIC MANAGEMENT

The treatment of breast cancer MC is multidisciplinary and should be discussed on a case-by-case basis in a multidisciplinary consultation meeting. Optimal management is based on the determination of prognostic factors, metastatic disease status, and patient preference. It has two components: local treatment of CD and control of systemic disease. It is based on RT, surgery and systemic therapy. Symptomatic treatment is essential, as it aims to reduce peri-tumor edema and prevent possible epileptic seizures. It consists of corticosteroid therapy, possibly associated with anticonvulsant treatment

4.1 Place of surgery:

The surgical intervention may consist of either open surgical resection of the brain lesion or a cerebrospinal fluid (CSF) shunt outside the central nervous system to decrease the intracerebral pressure secondary to the mass effect generated by the brain lesion exposing the patient to a risk of neurological deterioration and commitment[22]. The efficacy of surgical resection was demonstrated by Patchell et al, who randomized 48 patients with a single CD between the surgery followed by RT arm of the brain in toto and the needle biopsy followed by RT arm, finding a decrease in local recurrence rate in favor of the arm that includes surgical resection 20% vs 52% with $p<0.02$) as well as an improvement in overall survival (15 weeks Vs 40 weeks with $p<0.01$)[23]. However, this treatment option is reserved for patients in good general condition, with controlled metastatic disease and a number of CDs of 1 to 3 lesions. Norris et al reported in his study that patients who had 2 or 3 completely resected metastases had comparable therapeutic results to those operated for a single CD[24].

In a study by Mintz et al that randomized patients with CD (<4 lesions) between the surgery + EBRT arm and the EBRT alone arm, there was no survival benefit for patients with impaired general status or uncontrolled systemic disease[25].

Furthermore, the choice of surgical resection depends on the size of the brain lesion and its location. Surgery is not recommended if complete resection of the CD is not possible, the lesion is close to a functional area (eloquent area) or if the lesion is located in a deep area due to the increased risk of morbidity and significant neurological sequelae. Awake surgery has contributed to the resection of some CDs located in areas but it is not yet available in our country[26].

4.2 RT Place:

External encephalic radiotherapy (EER) or in toto encephalic radiotherapy has long been the standard treatment for CD. Studies since the 1980s have shown a benefit of EBRT at 30 Gy compared to EBRT at 20 Gy and supportive care. This benefit has been shown in terms of OS (3 to 6 months Vs 1 month) and complete or partial response with neurological symptom control of 30 to 60%. Several authors have retrospectively analyzed the response rates of MC in breast cancer to EBRT and found response rates of 65 to 82% and recurrence rates of 0 to 50%[27]

(Table 1)

Study	Year	Referenc e	Effect if	Number MC	RT Scheme	Response rate e(%)	Relapse rate (%)
Nieder et al	1997	[28]	46	Average :4	30Gy/1 0f	65	0
Ogura et al	2003	[29]	36	Multiple	30Gy/1 0f 50Gy/2 5f Boost : 10 cases	82	32
Mahmo ud Ahmed et al	2002	[30]	116	Unique :2 0 2-3 :28 4-9 : 50	30Gy/1 0f	NF	32
				>9 : 8			
The Scodan et al	2007	[30]	117	Multiple	30Gy/1 0f	NF	50

*Gy: Gray, f: Fraction

Table 1: Studies that evaluated the role of radiation therapy alone in patients with CD secondary to breast carcinoma

Some studies have looked at treatment regimens with different doses and fractions, concluding that the dose of 30 Gy in 10 fractions provides good results with good tolerance and the least neurological toxicity[27].

Stereotactic radiotherapy (SR) is a technique that consists of delivering several high-dose radiation beams in fractions with a reduced number of sessions in a predefined reduced volume (Figure 4, 5) [18].

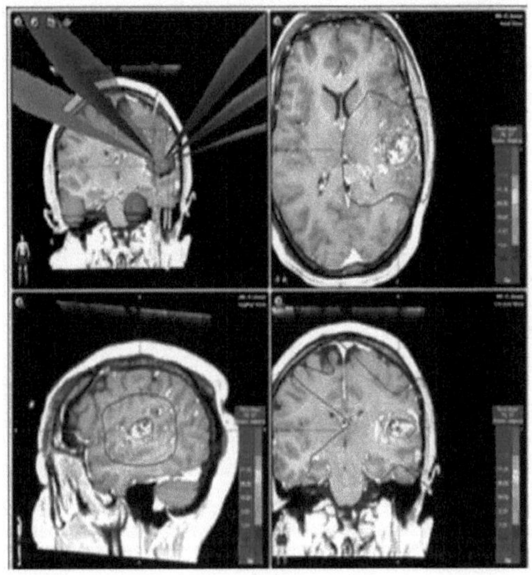

Figure 4: Dosimetry of an arteriovenous malformation

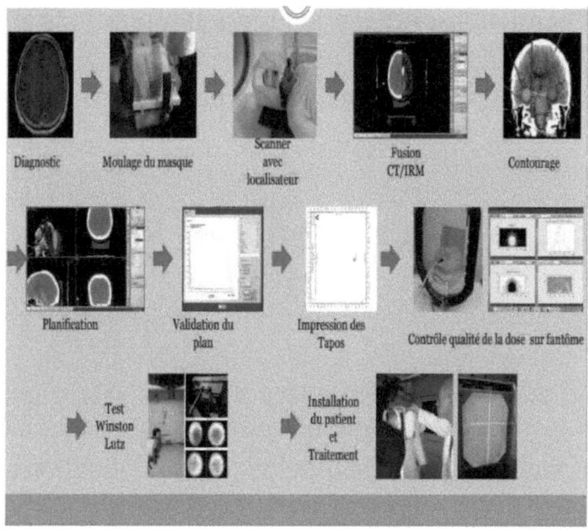

Figure 5: Stereotaxis procedure

SR is reserved for certain patients with 1 to 4 brain lesions of less than 3 cm in size at a deep location or close to an eloquent area, with an OS of more than 3 months and a preserved general state[32,33].

Several studies have compared SR plus EBRT versus EBRT alone and concluded that SR plus EBRT improves local disease control in the subgroups with less than 4 metastases, but this improvement has not been demonstrated in the subgroup with multiple metastases.

The benefit in terms of OS has also not been demonstrated[18,34].

SR has also been compared to surgical resection in several non-randomized studies.

There was no difference in local disease control but SR had the advantage of being non-invasive with less morbidity[35-37].

SR was not a technique available for the patients studied in our series.

4.4. Corticosteroid therapy:

Corticosteroid therapy helps to reduce the mass effect and peritumoral edema that is caused by CD and helps to alleviate clinical symptoms. The recommended dose is Dexamethasone at a dose of 4 to 8mg (or equivalent). Radiation therapy is started as soon as the diagnosis is made and continued throughout the course of the radiotherapy to reduce post-radiation oedema [38].

4.5. Place of systemic treatment:

The choice of systemic therapy depends on the patient's general condition, the status of the disease at the time of the onset of CD, the molecular characteristics of the primary tumor, and the different treatments previously received and the response they produced.The place of cytotoxic chemotherapy has been shown by several studies to improve survival in patients with multiple CD after EBRT[2,39,40]. However, the choice of the molecule for the treatment of CD is more difficult than for other metastatic sites because the chemotherapy must be able to cross the blood-brain barrier (BBB) and be present at effective concentrations in the CSF. Pitz et al reviewed ten studies evaluating the penetration of chemotherapy agents into brain metastases. The molecules and protocols that were evaluated included CMF, CAF, cisplatin, carboplatin, capecitabine, etoposide, anthracyclines and doxorubicineliposomal, temozolomide, irinotecan, methotrexate, taxanes, cyclophosphamide, navelbine, gemcitabine. Response rates to the different chemotherapy agents vary from 18 to 68% according to the different studies [41,42].

In an early series using multidrug therapies with cyclophosphamide, anthracyclines, 5-FU, methotrexate or vincristine, the response rates observed at the brain and systemic levels were similar and approached 50%, with 10% complete response[41].

Temozolomide, which diffuses well into the CNS but is only weakly active in breast cancer, did not show a significant response in patients with brain parenchymal metastases of breast cancer as a single agent[36].

Several retrospective series have reported complete and durable responses to capecitabine, including in heavily pretreated patients, with particularly long survival[41].

The role of hormone therapy has been demonstrated in disease control metastatic HR+ but its effect on MC has not been established. Tamoxifen and its metabolites can reach sufficient concentrations in the CSF, but responses to hormone therapy were not significant. This could be explained by the fact that MCs developed during known RH+ breast carcinomas may lose RH expression [44].

For MC in tumors with an overexpressed HER gene, patients treated with chemotherapy had better survival compared to patients who did not receive it (16.4 vs. 3.7 months). This was also observed in patients who received trastuzumab (Figure 5) (17.5 vs. 3.8 months)[45].

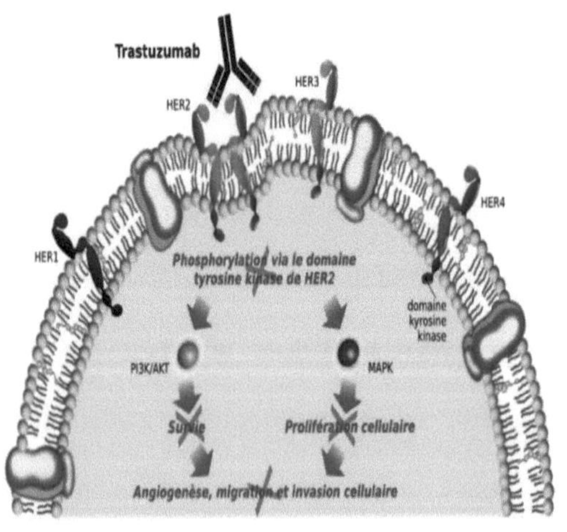

Figure 5: Mechanism of action of trastuzumab

There are no data in the literature on the use of pertuzumab (Figure6).

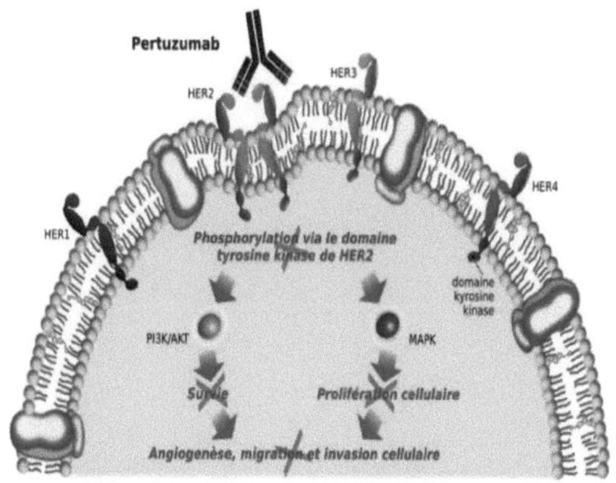

Figure 6: Mechanism of action of pertuzumab

Lapatinib is a specific enzyme inhibitor of receptor tyrosine kinase, EGFR and HER2.It is a small molecule whose pharmacological characteristics allow cerebral diffusion across the BBB and allow to consider its anti-tumor activity in this location.

Its action has been studied in combination with capecitabine in several studies in comparison to capecitabine alone.Petrelli et al in a review of the literature published in 2017, collected 12 studies that looked at the combination Lapatinib+ Capecitabine in MC during HER overexpressed breast carcinoma and concluded that this combination can be proposed for patients with cerebral progression after local treatment or when re-irradiation is not an option[46].

Lapatinib is not yet available in this country.

5. STUDY OF SURVIVAL AND PROGNOSTIC FACTORS

5.1 SG Study:

The occurrence of CD during breast carcinoma modifies the prognosis of the disease. In the series published in the literature, the average OS varies between 7.3 and 10.6 months [12,40-42].

In the series by Ben Kridis et al, the mean OS was 8 months in the MC subgroup secondary to breast carcinoma (Figure 7) [14].

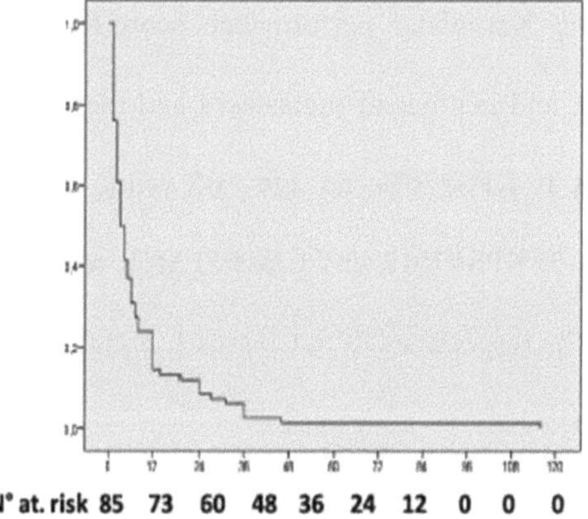

Figure 7: Overall survival of breast cancer with brain metastases

OS varies according to molecular classification and treatments administered. In the HER overexpressed subgroup, it can reach 2 to 3 years in patients treated with targeted therapy [43] but it remains very reduced in patients without access to this treatment and varies from 3.4 to 5.8 months which was found in our series (5.5 months). Triple-negative breast carcinomas always have a more guarded prognosis as brain progression is most often part of systemic disease progression in several metastatic sites. The mean OS ranged from 3 to 5.9 months [40-42].The RadiationTherapyOncology Group (RTOG) performed a prognostic analysis (Recursive partitioning analysis (RPA) and OS of MCs based on Karnofsky performance score(KPS), age, systemic disease status, and number of metastases and then divided them into classes: Class 1: KPS≥70%, an age >65 years, controlled systemic disease, Class 3: KPS<70%, and Class 2: MCs without the criteria of Class 1 or 3.The respective OS in Classes 1, 2 and 3 were 7.1, 4.1 and 2.3 months[44].

5.2 Study of prognostic factors:

Several prognostic factors influencing OS after the development of MC during breast carcinoma have been studied in the literature. Braccini et al found that the molecular biology of the primary tumor, the presence of extracranial metastases, RTOG RPA Class(Class 1 and 2 have a better prognosis)[51], local treatment and chemotherapy were prognostic factors influencing survival[47].

De Leso et al found the same results in addition to the WHO score and treatment with stereotactic radiotherapy [13].

Multivariate analysis in these studies retained that systemic treatment, local treatment, WHO score and RPA score were independently significant. On the other hand, Chow et al found only HR status as a significant prognostic factor and Li et al retained only histological grade and stage of the disease[52,53].

CONCLUSION

Breast cancer constitutes 15 to 20% of the etiologies of CD. CDs occur late in life, in the 5th decade.Their incidence has been increasing during the last decades thanks to the improvement of the global survival and the performance of the imaging techniques. A higher rate of recurrence of metastatic disease only as CD without progression of other metastatic sites has been seen in the literature especially in the HER overexpressed subgroup.Their clinical presentation is polymorphic, ranging from a headache to focal deficits or comitiality.MRI is the examination of choice in the diagnosis of CD and has allowed a better detection of multiple lesions and a better characterization of tumor lesions thanks to its different sequences, notably spectroscopy.The therapeutic management should be discussed in multidisciplinary consultation meetings on a case-by-case basis and the therapeutic strategy should be chosen according to the patient's general condition, the number and location of CDs and the status of metastatic disease.Local treatment with surgery or stereotactic radiotherapy is reserved for patients with a number of metastases <4 in patients with preserved general condition and controlled systemic disease.EBRT at a dose of 30Gy has long been an important pillar of treatment and has improved patient survival. In toto encephalic radiotherapy remains the reference treatment for brain metastases, especially in patients with multiple metastases or metastases too large to allow radiosurgery. This irradiation is also indicated in patients whose disease progresses after surgery or radiosurgery for brain metastases. The objective response rate for radiation therapy is approximately 60%. Radiosurgery is reserved for situations in which the metastases are limited in number (less than 4) and less than 3 cm in diameter, but are not accessible to surgerySystemic therapy has resulted in increased survival in patients with cerebral progression.The choice of the molecule depends on the previously prescribed treatments and its ability to pass through the BBB and to be at effective concentrations in the CNS.Multidrug therapies based on cyclophosphamide, anthracyclines, 5-FU, and methotrexate have resulted in response rates at the brain and systemic levels of 50%.Several retrospective series have reported complete and durable responses to capecitabine, including in heavily pretreated patients, with particularly long survival.The role of hormone therapy has been demonstrated in the control of RH+ metastatic disease but its effect on MC has not been established. Tamoxifen and its metabolites can reach sufficient concentrations in CSF but responses to hormone therapy have not been significant.In the HER-overexpressed subgroup, trastuzumab and lapatinib plus capecitabine are treatment options that have improved disease prognosis in this subgroup but are not yet available to our patients.There are currently no data to identify a group of patients at risk who would benefit from prophylactic radiation therapy.The triple negative subgroup has the most guarded prognosis.OS from the diagnosis of CD does not usually exceed 12 months, but may reach 2-3 years in HER-overexpressed patients who have been treated with targeted therapies.Prognostic factors influencing survival after diagnosis of CD described in the literature are:WHO score, molecular biology of the primary tumor, presence of extracranial metastases, RTOG RPA class, local treatment and chemotherapy.

REFERENCES

1. Cancer today [Internet]. [cited 3 Dec 2019]. Available from: http://gco.iarc.fr/today/home

2. Lee SS, Ahn J-H, Kim MK, Sym SJ, Gong G, Ahn SD, et al. Brain metastases in breast cancer: prognostic factors and management. Breast Cancer Res Treat. Oct 2008;111(3):523-30.

3. Weil RJ, Palmieri DC, Bronder JL, Stark AM, Steeg PS. Breast cancer metastasis to the central nervous system. Am J Pathol. 2005 Oct;167(4):913-20.

4. Rivoire M. Should synchronous metastases be differentiated from metastasesmetachronous ? :3.

5. Ben Kridis W, Toumi N, Ben Salah H, Sghaier S, Kammoun I, Boudawara Z, et al. Therapeutic results and prognostic factors of brain metastases from breast cancer: Single center experience. Breast J. 2019;25(4):778-80.

6. Tabouret E, Bauchet L, Carpentier AF. Brain metastases epidemiology and biology. Bull Cancer (Paris). jan 2013;100(1):57-62.

7. Kirsch DG, Loeffler JS. Brain metastases in patients with breast cancer: new horizons. Clin Breast Cancer. June 2005;6(2):115-24.

8. Boogerd W, Vos VW, Hart AA, Baris G. Brain metastases in breast cancer; natural history, prognostic factors and outcome. J Neurooncol. Feb 1993;15(2):165-74.

9. Tsukada Y, Fouad A, Pickren JW, Lane WW. Central nervous system metastasis from breast carcinoma. Autopsy study. Cancer. 15 Dec 1983;52(12):2349-54.

10. Yau T, Swanton C, Chua S, Sue A, Walsh G, Rostom A, et al. Incidence, pattern and timing of brain metastases among patients with advanced breast cancer treated with trastuzumab. Acta Oncol Stockh Swed. 2006;45(2):196-201.

11. Witzel I, Kantelhardt EJ, Milde-Langosch K, Ihnen M, Zeitz J, Harbeck N, et al. Management of patients with brain metastases receiving trastuzumab treatment for metastatic breast cancer. Onkologie. 2011;34(6):304-8.

12. Kaplan MA, Isikdogan A, Koca D, Kucukoner M, Gumusay O, Yildiz R, et al. Biological subtypes and survival outcomes in breast cancer patients with brain metastases (study of the Anatolian Society

of Medical Oncology). Oncology. 2012;83(3):141-50.

13. De Ieso PB, Schick U, Rosenfelder N, Mohammed K, Ross GM. Breast cancer brain metastases - A 12 year review of treatment outcomes. The Breast. august 2015;24(4):426-33.

14. Ben Kridis W, Toumi N, Ben Salah H, Sghaier S, Kammoun I, Boudawara Z, Daoud J, Khanfir A, Frikha M. Therapeutic results and prognostic factors of brain metastases from breast cancer: Single center experience. Breast J. 2019 Jul;25(4):778-780.

15. Barnholtz-Sloan JS, Sloan AE, Davis FG, Vigneau FD, Lai P, Sawaya RE. Incidence proportions of brain metastases in patients diagnosed (1973 to 2001) in the Metropolitan Detroit Cancer Surveillance System. J Clin Oncol Off J Am Soc Clin Oncol. 15 Jul 2004;22(14):2865-72.

16. Bowman KM, Kumthekar P. Medical management of brain metastases and leptomeningeal disease in patients with breast carcinoma. Future Oncol Lond Engl. Feb 2018;14(4):391-407.

17. Olson EM, Abdel-Rasoul M, Maly J, Wu CS, Lin NU, Shapiro CL. Incidence and risk of central nervous system metastases as site of first recurrence in patients with HER2-positive breast cancer treated

with adjuvant trastuzumab. Ann Oncol Off J Eur Soc Med Oncol. June 2013;24(6):1526-33.

18. Ewend MG, Morris DE, Carey LA, Ladha AM, Brem S. Guidelines for the initial management of metastatic brain tumors: role of surgery, radiosurgery, and radiation therapy. J Natl Compr Cancer Netw JNCCN. May 2008;6(5):505-13; quiz 514.

19. Saha A, Ghosh S, Roy C, Choudhury K, Chakrabarty B, Sarkar R. Demographic and clinical profile of patients with brain metastases: A retrospective study. Asian J Neurosurg. 2013;8(3):157.

20. POPE WB. Brain metastases: neuroimaging. Handb Clin Neurol. 2018;149:89-112.

21. Naggara O, Brami-Zylberberg F, Rodrigo S, Raynal M, Meary E, Godon-Hardy S, et al. Imaging of intracranial metastases in adults. J Radiol. June 2006;87(6):792-806.

22. Soffietti R, Abacioglu U, Baumert B, Combs SE, Kinhult S, Kros JM, et al. Diagnosis and treatment of brain metastases from solid tumors: guidelines from the European Association of Neuro-Oncology (EANO). Neuro-Oncol. 01 2017;19(2):162-74.

23. Patchell RA, Tibbs PA, Walsh JW, Dempsey RJ, Maruyama Y, Kryscio RJ, et al. A Randomized Trial of Surgery in the Treatment of Single Metastases to the Brain. N Engl J Med. Feb 22, 1990;322(8):494-500.

24. Norris LK, Grossman SA, Olivi A. Neoplastic meningitis following surgical resection of isolated cerebellar metastasis: a potentially preventable complication. J Neurooncol. May 1997;32(3):215-23.

25. Mintz AH, Kestle J, Rathbone MP, Gaspar L, Hugenholtz H, Fisher B, et al. A randomized trial to assess the efficacy of surgery in addition to radiotherapy in patients with a single cerebral metastasis. Cancer. 1 Oct 1996;78(7):1470-6.

26. Chua TH, See AAQ, Ang BT, King NKK. Awake Craniotomy for Resection of Brain Metastases: A Systematic Review. World Neurosurg. dec 2018;120:e1128-35.

27. Tallet AV, Azria D, Le Rhun E, Barlesi F, Carpentier AF, Gonçalves A, et al. Rationale for the use of upfront whole brain irradiation in patients with brain metastases from breast cancer. Int J Mol Sci. May 8, 2014;15(5):8138-52.

28. Nieder C, Berberich W, Schnabel K. Tumor-related prognostic factors for remission of brain metastases after radiotherapy. Int J Radiat Oncol Biol Phys. 1 August 1997;39(1):25-30.

29. Ogura M, Mitsumori M, Okumura S, Yamauchi C, Kawamura S, Oya N, et al. Radiation therapy for brain metastases from breast cancer. Breast Cancer Tokyo Jpn. 2003;10(4):349-55.

30. Mahmoud-Ahmed AS, Suh JH, Lee S-Y, Crownover RL, Barnett GH. Results of whole brain radiotherapy in patients with brain metastases from breast cancer: a retrospective study. Int J Radiat Oncol Biol Phys. 2002 Nov 1;54(3):810-7.

31. Le Scodan R, Massard C, Mouret-Fourme E, Guinebretierre JM, Cohen-Solal C, De Lalande B, et al. Brain metastases from breast carcinoma: validation of the radiation therapy oncology group recursive partitioning analysis classification and proposition of a new prognostic score. Int J Radiat Oncol Biol Phys. 1 Nov 2007;69(3):839-45.

32. Khalsa SSS, Chinn M, Krucoff M, Sherman JH. The role of stereotactic radiosurgery for multiple brain metastases in stable systemic disease: a review of the literature. Acta Neurochir (Wien). july 2013;155(7):1321-7; discussion 1327-1328.

33. Mehta MP, Tsao MN, Whelan TJ, Morris DE, Hayman JA, Flickinger JC, et al. The American Society for Therapeutic Radiology and Oncology (ASTRO) evidence-based review of the role of radiosurgery for brain metastases. Int J Radiat Oncol Biol Phys. 2005 Sep 1;63(1):37-46.

34. Rades D, Huttenlocher S, Hornung D, Blanck O, Schild SE, Fischer D. Do patients with very few brain metastases from breast cancer benefit from whole-brain radiotherapy in addition to radiosurgery? Radiat Oncol Lond Engl [Internet]. 4 Dec 2014 [cited 14 Dec 2019];9. Available from: https://www.ncbi.nlm.nih.gov/pmc/articles/PMC4265339/

35. Muacevic A, Wowra B, Siefert A, Tonn J-C, Steiger H-J, Kreth FW. Microsurgery plus whole brain irradiation versus Gamma Knife surgery alone for treatment of single metastases to the brain: a randomized controlled multicentre phase III trial. J Neurooncol. May 2008;87(3):299-307.

36. Sneed PK, Suh JH, Goetsch SJ, Sanghavi SN, Chappell R, Buatti JM, et al. A multi-institutional review of radiosurgery alone vs. radiosurgery with whole brain radiotherapy as the initial management of brain metastases. Int J Radiat Oncol Biol Phys. 1 Jul

2002;53(3):519-26.

37. Regine WF, Huhn JL, Patchell RA, St Clair WH, Strottmann J, Meigooni A, et al. Risk of symptomatic brain tumor recurrence and neurologic deficit after radiosurgery alone in patients with newly diagnosed brain metastases: results and implications. Int J Radiat Oncol Biol Phys. Feb 1, 2002;52(2):333-8.

38. Ryken TC, McDermott M, Robinson PD, Ammirati M, Andrews DW, Asher AL, et al. The role of steroids in the management of brain metastases: a systematic review and evidence-based clinical practice guideline. J Neurooncol. Jan 2010;96(1):103-14.

39. Kim H-J, Im S-A, Keam B, Kim Y-J, Han S-W, Kim TM, et al. Clinical outcome of central nervous system metastases from breast cancer: differences in survival depending on systemic treatment. J Neurooncol. jan 2012;106(2):303-13.

40. Lagerwaard FJ, Levendag PC, Nowak PJ, Eijkenboom WM, Hanssens PE, Schmitz PI. Identification of prognostic factors in patients with brain metastases: a review of 1292 patients. Int J Radiat Oncol Biol Phys. March 1, 1999;43(4):795-803.

41. Bachelot T, Le Rhun É, Labidi-Gally I, Heudel P, Gilabert M, Bonneterre J, et al. Systemic treatment of brain metastases from breast cancer: cytotoxic chemotherapy and targeted therapies. Bull Cancer (Paris). jan 2013;100(1):7-14.

42. Pitz MW, Desai A, Grossman SA, Blakeley JO. Tissue concentration of systemically administered antineoplastic agents in human brain tumors. J Neurooncol. sept 2011;104(3):629-38.

43. Abrey LE, Olson JD, Raizer JJ, Mack M, Rodavitch A, Boutros DY, et al. A phase II trial of temozolomide for patients with recurrent or progressive brain metastases. J Neurooncol. July 2001;53(3):259-65.

44. Liu MC, Cortés J, O'Shaughnessy J. Challenges in the treatment of hormone receptor-positive, HER2-negative metastatic breast cancer with brain metastases. Cancer Metastasis Rev. June 2016;35(2):323-32.

45. Shah N, Mohammad AS, Saralkar P, Sprowls SA, Vickers SD, John D, et al. Investigational chemotherapy and novel pharmacokinetic mechanisms for the treatment of breast cancer brain metastases. Pharmacol Res. June 2018;132:47-68.

46. Petrelli F, Ghidini M, Lonati V, Tomasello G, Borgonovo K, Ghilardi M, et al. The efficacy of lapatinib and capecitabine in HER-2 positive breast cancer with brain metastases: A systematic review and pooled analysis. Eur J Cancer Oxf Engl 1990. 2017;84:141-8.

47. Braccini AL, Azria D, Thezenas S, Romieu G, Ferrero JM, Jacot W. Prognostic factors of brain metastases from breast cancer: impact of targeted therapies. Breast Edinb Scotl. Oct 2013;22(5):993-8.

48. Niwinska A, Murawska M, Pogoda K. Breast cancer brain metastases: differences in survival depending on biological subtype, RPA RTOG prognostic class and systemic treatment after whole-brain radiotherapy (WBRT). Ann Oncol. 2010 May 1;21(5):942-8.

49. Niikura N, Hayashi N, Masuda N, Takashima S, Nakamura R, Watanabe K, et al. Treatment outcomes and prognostic factors for patients with brain metastases from breast cancer of each subtype: a multicenter retrospective analysis. Breast Cancer Res Treat. August 2014;147(1):103-12.

50. McKee MJ, Keith K, Deal AM, Garrett AL, Wheless AA, Green RL, et al. A Multidisciplinary Breast Cancer Brain Metastases Clinic: The University of North Carolina Experience. The Oncologist. jan 2016;21(1):16-20.

51. Gaspar L, Scott C, Rotman M, Asbell S, Phillips T, Wasserman T, et al. Recursive partitioning analysis (RPA) of prognostic factors in three radiation therapy oncology group (RTOG) brain metastases trials. Int J Radiat Oncol. March 1997;37(4):745-51.

52. Chow L, Suen D, Ma KK, Kwong A. Identifying risk factors for brain metastasis in breast cancer patients: Implication for a vigorous surveillance program. Asian J Surg. Oct 2015;38(4):220-3.

53. Li R, Zhang K, Siegal GP, Wei S. Clinicopathological factors associated with survival in patients with breast cancer brain metastasis. Hum Pathol. 2017;64:53-60.

TABLE OF CONTENTS

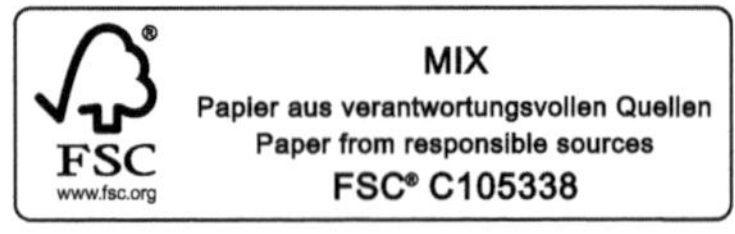

Printed by Books on Demand GmbH, Norderstedt / Germany